Bariatric Surgery

(Weight Loss Surgery)

All You Need to Know

Dr. Sheila Harrison

Disclaimer

This content serves to provide general information about the disease and aims to empower you to seek prompt medical assistance if necessary to prevent complications. It's essential to stress that this information is not a substitute for consulting a qualified physician. The field of medical science is continually evolving, and due to the dynamic nature of medical knowledge, we recommend seeking expert advice if you encounter any inconsistencies or intend to take action based on the information in this content. Never disregard professional medical guidance or delay treatment based on something you've read online, including this material, or from any other online source. Always remember that the internet cannot cure you; rather, healing comes through the guidance of medical professionals and the providence of God.

Table of Content

Section 1

Bariatric surgery

Bariatric surgery, often known as weight loss surgery, is a medical treatment performed on people who are obese and have not lost weight using traditional techniques such as diet and exercise. There are several types of bariatric surgery that doctors recommend on an individual basis. The surgery's goal is to assist patients in achieving considerable and long-term weight loss. Weight loss can enhance their overall health and quality of life.

Bariatric surgery is typically performed in hospitals or surgical centers by qualified surgeons with weight reduction surgery training. They do this surgery while under general anesthesia.

Types of Surgical Techniques Employed

Doctors select particular surgical procedures based on the type of bariatric surgery being performed.

Among the most prevalent techniques are:

- **Laparoscopic surgery:** The method is non-invasive. Small incisions in the abdomen are made for laparoscopic surgery. To execute the surgery, the surgeons employ sophisticated surgical instruments as well as a camera. Laparoscopic surgery speeds up healing by reducing recovery time, bleeding, incision size, pain, and scars.

- **Open surgery:** Laparotomy, often known as open surgery, is performed by making a wide incision in the abdomen. During laparotomy, a surgeon frequently forms a small pouch in the stomach and reroutes the small intestine to this pouch, bypassing portion of the stomach and small intestine. This limits the quantity of food the patient can ingest and absorb, causing weight loss.

Patients are usually admitted to the hospital for a few days after surgery to heal before being discharged. To evaluate progress and give continuous assistance, follow-up meetings with the surgeon and other healthcare experts will be required.

When is bariatric surgery recommended?

Individuals with a BMI of 40 or higher may be advised to undergo bariatric surgery. They may also advise surgery for anyone with a BMI of 35 or higher and at least one obesity-related health problem. Type 2 diabetes, high blood pressure, sleep apnea, and joint difficulties are all obesity-related illnesses. Individuals with a BMI between 30 and 35 may potentially benefit from bariatric surgery, according to doctors. Individuals in these circumstances must have serious health problems as a result of their obesity and have failed to achieve and sustain weight loss through other means.

When alternative treatments of weight loss have failed to achieve and maintain weight loss, bariatric surgery may be advised. Diet and exercise are two weight loss techniques. The operation can result in significant weight loss and the improvement or resolution of obesity-related health issues. It is critical to understand that bariatric surgery is a major procedure. It should only be considered after all other weight loss procedures have been tried and failed.

Each instance, however, is unique. You should check with a healthcare expert before deciding to have bariatric surgery. Only qualified doctors can analyze the risks and advantages depending on individual factors, which is critical.

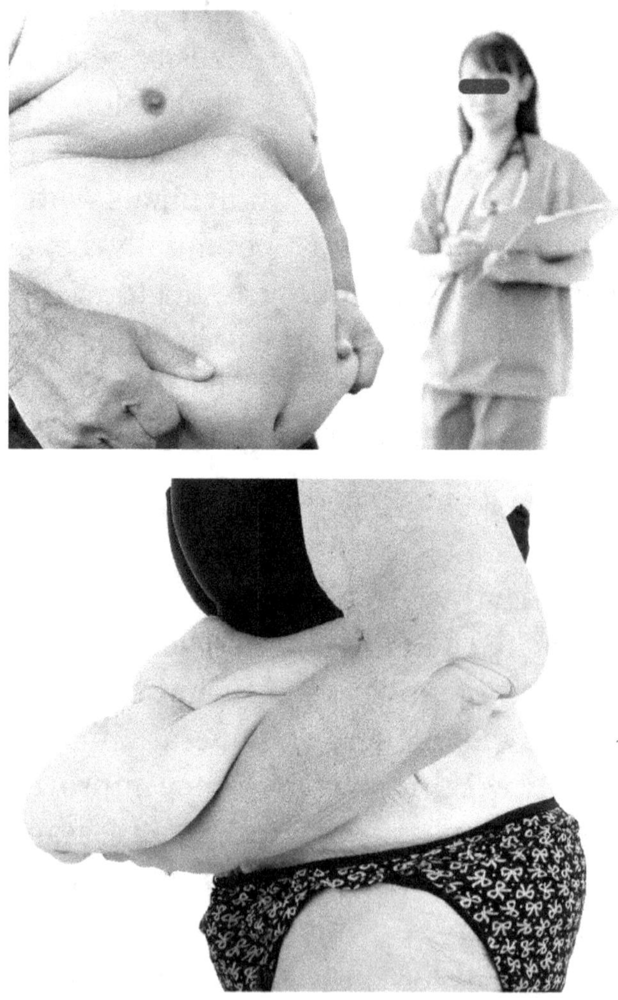

Section 2

The Various Types of Bariatric Surgery

Bariatric surgery is classified into numerous categories. Gastric bypass, sleeve gastrectomy, adjustable gastric banding, and biliopancreatic diversion with a duodenal switch are all part of the procedure. Each of the methods takes an own approach to weight loss.

The following are the most prevalent types of bariatric surgery:

- **Gastric Bypass Surgery:** Bariatric surgery includes gastric bypass surgery. It entails developing a tiny stomach pouch. The small intestine is then rerouted to this pouch by the surgeon. This avoids the majority of the stomach and upper small intestine. As a result, the patient's capacity to eat meals at one time is reduced. The bypass made by the surgeon during gastric bypass surgery also influences nutrient absorption. This technique is often performed laparoscopically by surgeons. They achieve this by making small incisions in the abdomen. The treatment is carried out using a tiny camera and surgical equipment.

- **Sleeve Gastrectomy:** Another type of bariatric surgery is a sleeve gastrectomy. In a sleeve gastrectomy, the surgeon removes a major part of the stomach. This results in a more compact, banana-shaped stomach. This restricts the amount of food that can be eaten at one time. The hunger hormone ghrelin is also reduced with a sleeve gastrectomy, which can aid in appetite management.

- **Adjustable gastric banding:** Weight loss surgery of this type is known as adjustable gastric banding. A silicone band is wrapped around the top section of the stomach during adjustable gastric banding. This process results in the stomach being divided into two uneven portions. The upper portion functions as a replacement stomach, limiting food intake and aiding weight loss. Adjusting the band involves injecting or withdrawing fluid through a tiny channel under the skin.

- **Biliopancreatic diversion with duodenal switch:** BPD/DS (biliopancreatic diversion with duodenal switch) is a type of weight loss surgery that consists of two surgeries. The initial step in biliopancreatic diversion is to remove a big piece of the stomach. This results in a smaller, tubular-shaped stomach. The second step in the biliopancreatic diversion technique is to reroute the small intestine to the new stomach.

This is accomplished by bypassing much of the small intestine and reattaching it further down the intestine. It has the effect of limiting the amount of food that patients can consume. Biliopancreatic diversion reduces the absorption of calories and nutrients from diet. Medical specialists believe BPD/DS to be a difficult surgery. It is not as frequent as other types of weight loss surgery. Gastric bypass and sleeve gastrectomy are two examples of such procedures.

It is critical to consult with a knowledgeable healthcare expert about the dangers and advantages of BPD/DS. This is done to see if it's a good fit for a person's weight loss objectives and health demands.

- **Intragastric Balloon:** The intragastric balloon is a non-surgical and minimally invasive weight loss technique that includes inserting a deflated silicone balloon through the mouth into the stomach and filling it with saline solution. The balloon occupies stomach space. This produces a full feeling and limits the amount of food that may be consumed. This surgery is normally performed under anesthesia by surgeons and takes around 20-30 minutes. After six months, the balloon is removed. Long-term success necessitates lifestyle adjustments such as nutrition and exercise. Doctors usually believe that this technique is safe.

However, there are hazards and consequences to consider, such as nausea, vomiting, and balloon deflation. These treatments differ in their operation but they serve the same aim. Their purpose is to reduce stomach size or the body's ability to absorb meals. The technique chosen will be determined by a number of factors, including the patient's medical history, body mass index (BMI), and personal preferences. To identify the appropriate course of action for particular circumstances, it is critical to consult with a certified healthcare expert.

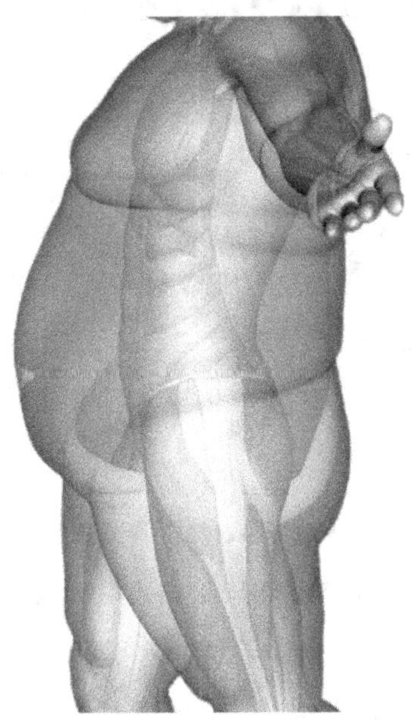

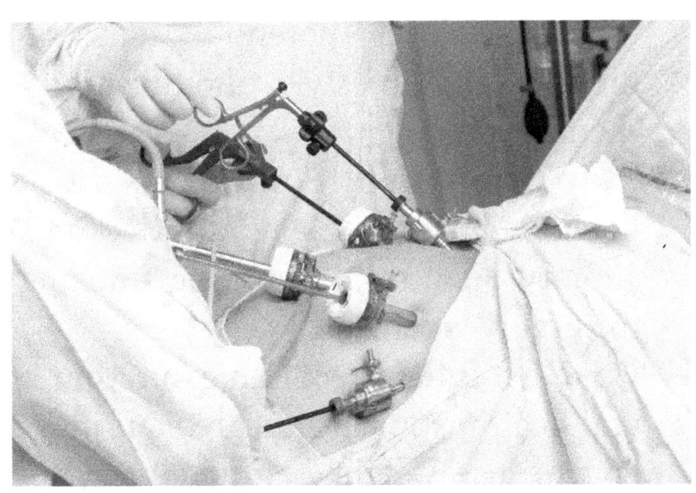

Section 3

How to prepare for bariatric surgery

Getting ready for bariatric surgery entails a number of steps to ensure that you are both physically and emotionally prepared for the procedure. Here are some general preparation tips:

- **Meet with your healthcare team:** You must consult with your surgeon, a registered dietitian, and possibly other medical professionals. It is critical that you discuss the procedure, potential dangers, and dietary and lifestyle modifications with them.
- **Stop smoking:** Smoking increases the likelihood of problems during and after surgery. As a result, quitting smoking prior to surgery is critical.
- **Lose weight:** Depending on your weight and health, your healthcare staff may advise you to lose weight before surgery to lower the chance of complications.

- **Follow a special diet:** Before bariatric surgery, your dietician will most likely give you a specific diet to follow in order to prepare your body for the treatment and lower the size of your liver.
- **Attend instructional classes:** Many bariatric surgery programs provide educational workshops to help patients learn about the procedure, the recovery process, and the essential lifestyle modifications for long-term success.
- **Change your lifestyle:** This surgery is not a quick treatment for weight loss. To be successful, bariatric surgery necessitates considerable lifestyle adjustments. You may need to start exercising frequently, stop smoking, and make dietary modifications.
- **Address emotional health:** Bariatric surgery can have a substantial influence on emotional health, therefore any emotional concerns that may develop must be addressed. In this sense, support groups, counseling, and other resources can be beneficial.

Section 4

Risk Factors Associated with Bariatric Surgery

Bariatric surgery, like any other operation, has some risks and concerns. The following are some of the hazards linked with bariatric surgery:

- **Bleeding:** During or after bariatric surgery, there is a danger of bleeding, which may necessitate a blood transfusion.

- **Infection:** IInfection is a possibility with any surgery. Antibiotics may be required to treat an infection in some circumstances.

- **Blood clots:** In rare circumstances, blood clots can occur in the legs following bariatric surgery. Medication and early mobilization can help prevent them.

- **Leakage:** Surgical site leakage is possible, especially following gastric bypass surgery. Infection, sepsis, and other problems may result.

- **Malnutrition:** Malnutrition can result with bariatric surgery, especially if the patient does not follow an appropriate diet after surgery.

- **Dumping syndrome:** Dumping syndrome can occur in some cases of gastric bypass surgery. When food passes too quickly from the stomach and into the small intestine, it is spilled into the small intestine. Nausea, vomiting, diarrhea, and stomach cramps are all possible symptoms.

- **Gallstones:** Because of changes in bile acid circulation after bariatric surgery, rapid weight loss can increase the risk of developing gallstones.

- **Stricture:** After bariatric surgery, anastomotic stenosis, or narrowing of the stomach or intestine, can occur, resulting in blockages.

- **Hernia:** A hernia can develop at the incision site or in the abdominal wall.

Before making a decision, it is critical to examine the risks and benefits of bariatric surgery with a skilled healthcare expert. In many cases, the benefits of the procedure outweigh the risks, especially for those who are severely obese and have tried everything else to lose weight.

Section 5

Recovering after Bariatric Surgery

The recovery from bariatric surgery includes both physical and emotional rehabilitation. Here are some general pointers to assist you in your recovery following surgery:

- **Follow your doctor's directions:** It is critical to carefully follow your doctor's instructions for a proper recovery after bariatric surgery, including taking any recommended medications, attending follow-up appointments, and adhering to food and activity recommendations.

- **Increase physical activity gradually:** You should begin moving as soon as possible after surgery. You should, however, avoid heavy activity for many weeks after surgery. Because physical exercise is a crucial part of the recovery process after bariatric surgery, your doctor will give you specific advice on when and how to begin exercising again.

- **Focus on nutrition:** Following bariatric surgery, you will need to adhere to a strict diet in order to promote optimal healing and recuperation and to achieve maximum weight loss. Your doctor or a trained dietitian can advise you on what meals to consume, how much to eat, and how frequently to eat them.

- **Stay hydrated:** To minimize dehydration, it is critical to drink enough of fluids following surgery. Dehydration might impede your recovery after bariatric surgery. Your doctor will advise you on how much fluid to drink and what sorts of fluids to drink.

- **Take care of your incisions:** To avoid infection, keep the incision sites clean and dry. Your doctor will offer you detailed advice on how to care for the incisions so that you can recuperate from the bariatric surgery as soon as possible.

- **Address emotional health:** Bariatric surgery can have a substantial influence on emotional health, therefore any emotional concerns that may develop must be addressed. Support groups, therapy, and other tools can be beneficial during the bariatric surgery recovery process.

- **Please be patient:** Weight loss with bariatric surgery is usually slow. Significant outcomes may take several months. It is critical to be patient and to concentrate on creating long-term lifestyle improvements.

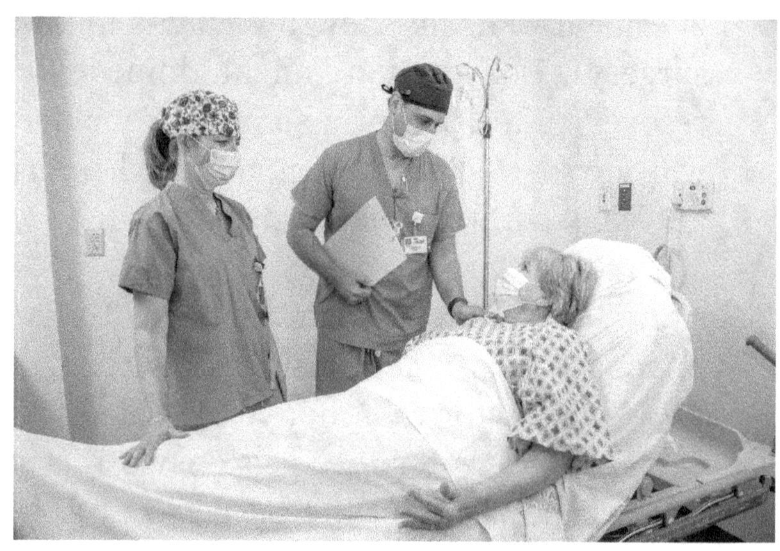

Section 6
Life After Bariatric Surgery

After bariatric surgery, life can be both pleasant and difficult. The procedure can help you lose weight and improve various health concerns, but it also necessitates considerable lifestyle modifications to ensure long-term success. Here are some general pointers for adjusting to life after bariatric surgery:

- **Follow the advice of your medical team:** Your healthcare team will give you particular instructions for food, exercise, and post-surgery care. It is critical to follow these instructions in order to achieve long-term success and avoid difficulties.

- **Eat a nutritious diet:** To promote good recovery and weight loss after bariatric surgery, you will need to follow a specialized diet. Your doctor or a trained dietitian can advise you on what meals to consume, how much to eat, and how frequently to eat them.

- **Stay active:** Regular physical activity is essential for weight loss and overall health. Your healthcare staff can advise you on when and how to begin exercising again after surgery.

- **Attend follow-up appointments:** Regular follow-up appointments with your healthcare team are important to monitor your progress and adjust your treatment plan as needed.

- **Be patient:** Weight loss after bariatric surgery is typically gradual, and it may take several months to see significant results. It is important to be patient and to focus on making sustainable lifestyle changes.

- **Adjust to a new lifestyle:** Bariatric surgery requires significant lifestyle changes, including changes to diet, exercise, and self-care. It is important to adjust to this new lifestyle and develop habits that will support long-term success.

Section 7

Advantages and Disadvantages of Bariatric Surgery

Bariatric surgery can result in long-term weight loss and the resolution of obesity-related illnesses. However, it comes with surgical risks, nutritional inadequacies, and psychological problems, so individuals must measure the benefits against the potential drawbacks before proceeding with the operation.

Bariatric surgery is becoming more popular as a realistic option for people who are severely obese. This surgical surgery tries to facilitate weight loss by reducing stomach size or modifying the structure of the digestive system. In this post, we will look at the benefits and drawbacks of bariatric surgery.

Advantages of Bariatric Surgery

Here are some of the possible advantages of bariatric surgery:

- **Weight loss that lasts:** Bariatric surgery allows for large and long-term weight loss. Weight loss as a result of bariatric surgery improves health outcomes, lowers the risk of obesity-related diseases, and improves overall quality of life.

- **Resolution of comorbid medical disorders:** Many people who have bariatric surgery see significant improvement or complete resolution of obesity-related diseases. High blood pressure, sleep apnea, and joint pain are examples of these conditions. PCOS may benefit from bariatric surgery as well. This can lead to less reliance on drugs and improved long-term health prospects. Type 2 diabetes may also benefit from bariatric surgery.

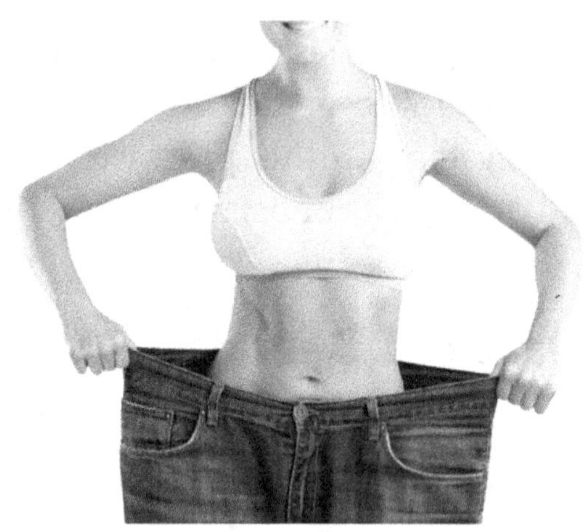

Disadvantages of bariatric surgery

The following are some of the potential disadvantages and dangers linked with bariatric surgery:

- **Surgical Risks:** Bariatric surgery, like any surgical procedure, has inherent risks. These dangers include the chance of infection, hemorrhage, blood clots, and anesthetic responses. The likelihood of such dangers occurring is low. However, it is critical to discuss them openly with a healthcare expert.

- **Deficiencies in Nutrition:** Bariatric surgery might impair the body's ability to absorb certain nutrients. To prevent deficits, this may demand lifetime vitamin and mineral supplementation. To maintain adequate nutritional status, regular monitoring and adherence to dietary requirements are required.

- **Psychological and emotional factors:** Weight loss from bariatric surgery can have a substantial impact on an individual's body image and self-esteem. Adapting to physical changes and developing a healthy relationship with food may necessitate continual psychological support and counseling.

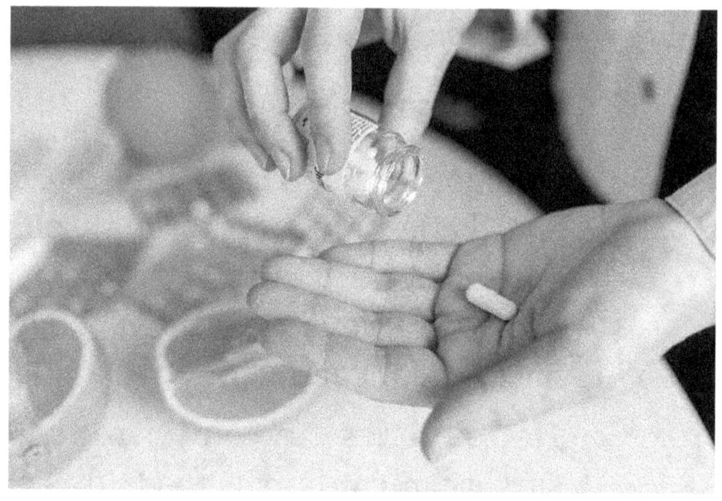

Deficiency supplement

Section 8

Reversal of Bariatric surgery

Bariatric surgery is typically seen as a permanent procedure. However, there are some circumstances in which bariatric surgery can be reversed.

- **Gastric Banding:** Gastric banding is possibly reversible bariatric surgery in which the surgeon puts an adjustable band around the stomach. A surgeon can remove the band surgically, returning the stomach to its natural size. However, you should be aware that removing the gastric band does not guarantee that you will regain your pre-surgery weight or health status.

- **Gastric Bypass:** Gastric bypass is a surgical treatment that alters the anatomy of the digestive system. Reversing gastric bypass is a technically difficult procedure that is frequently not suggested due to potential complications and low success rates. Reversal techniques may include reverting surgical alterations to their original form, although they are riskier and may not produce the desired results.

Considering Factors for Bariatric Surgery Reversal

Reversing bariatric surgery necessitates a team of medical specialists' thorough study and consideration of various issues. The operation itself has an impact on one's quality of life. The following are some of the factors that doctors consider:

- **Individual Circumstances:** Reversal choices are determined by a variety of situations. These include the precise bariatric procedure used, the patient's overall health, and the reasons for wanting the procedure reversed. It is critical to examine the feasibility and potential hazards with a healthcare practitioner who specializes in bariatric surgery.

- **Weight Control:** Reversing bariatric surgery does not ensure a return to pre-surgical weight. Individuals considering reversal should have a weight-management strategy in place, as well as a plan for resolving any underlying concerns that led to the initial operation.

- **Emotional and psychological well-being:** Having bariatric surgery reversed can have emotional and psychological consequences. It is critical to have enough support mechanisms in place. Counseling is also recommended to help manage the potential influence on body image, self-esteem, and mental well-being.

Finally, doctors often consider bariatric surgery to be a permanent procedure, with only certain forms, such as gastric banding, theoretically reversible. Reversing more invasive operations, such as gastric bypass, carries greater risks and may not produce the desired results. In rare situations, the surgery can result in death. A consultation with a healthcare practitioner who specializes in bariatric surgery is required to investigate your alternatives and make an informed decision.

Section 9

Before undergoing Bariatric Surgery, ask your doctor these questions.

You must understand that each case is unique, and a doctor is the best person to choose the best course of action. If you are considering bariatric surgery, you should ask your doctor many key questions to help you make an informed decision. If your doctor offers bariatric surgery, ask him the following questions:

What are the advantages and disadvantages of bariatric surgery?
Each surgery is distinct from the next. It is critical to understand the surgery's potential dangers and side effects, as well as the expected benefits in terms of weight loss and health improvements. So, talk to your doctor about it and make sure you understand the potential benefits and risks.

What kind of bariatric surgery is suggested for me?

Based on your medical history, body mass index (BMI), and personal preferences, your doctor can advise you on the best form of bariatric surgery for you.

What is the anticipated weight loss following surgery?

Weight loss expectations differ depending on the type of surgery, so having a realistic grasp of what to expect is essential.

How is the recuperation process?

You should be aware of the rehabilitation process, including the length of the hospital stay, the amount of time off work required, and any limits on physical activity or food.

What are the long-term goals and requirements following surgery?

Bariatric surgery is a long-term commitment, and it is critical to understand what modifications will be needed to maintain weight loss and manage any health concerns.

What are the dietary needs following surgery?

After surgery, you will most likely need to make substantial dietary adjustments, so it is critical to understand what foods you can and cannot eat, as well as any supplements that may be required.

What is the post-surgery support system like?

After surgery, it is critical to have a support system in place, including access to healthcare specialists, support groups, and counseling services.

These are just a few of the things you should ask your doctor before having bariatric surgery. It is critical to have an open and honest discussion with your healthcare professional in order to completely understand the risks and advantages of the procedure and make an informed decision.

Conclusion

To summarize, bariatric surgery can be a life-changing choice for people suffering from severe obesity and related health problems. It provides long-term weight loss as well as the possibility of resolving associated medical conditions. Despite this, there are hazards, such as surgical problems, nutritional deficits, and the need for ongoing psychological assistance. Before deciding on bariatric surgery, it is best to visit with a healthcare professional to determine candidacy and thoroughly weigh the advantages and cons based on specific circumstances.

FAQ on Bariatric Surgery

Is there any effect of bariatric surgery on renal health?

Although bariatric surgery does not directly address kidney health, it may have indirect advantages. Obesity and certain weight-related diseases might contribute to renal issues. Bariatric surgery may reduce some risk factors related to renal disease by facilitating weight loss and increasing general health.

Is bariatric surgery beneficial to diabetes management?

Yes. Diabetes patients can benefit tremendously from bariatric surgery by improving their condition management. The procedure frequently results in significant weight loss, which can lead to better blood sugar management and less dependency on diabetic medication.

Does bariatric surgery have an effect on liver health?

Bariatric surgery has been shown to improve liver health. It has been shown to be beneficial in the treatment of non-alcoholic fatty liver disease

(NAFLD) and non-alcoholic steatohepatitis (NASH). Weight loss as a result of the operation can aid in the reduction of liver fat and inflammation.

How can bariatric surgery affect patients' cholesterol levels?

In terms of lowering elevated cholesterol levels, bariatric surgery has shown promising outcomes. The technique may contribute to weight loss and changes in metabolic functioning, resulting in lower levels of LDL cholesterol (often referred to as 'bad' cholesterol) and higher levels of HDL cholesterol (usually referred to as 'good' cholesterol).

How can bariatric surgery affect bone health?

Bariatric surgery can have an impact on bone health, especially in obese people. Rapid weight loss after surgery may raise the risk of bone density loss and calcium deficiency. However, the impact on bone health can be reduced with correct supervision and post-surgery care, including vitamin and mineral prescription, exercise, and a balanced diet.

Is it possible to get pregnant after having bariatric surgery?

Weight loss via surgery may enhance reproductive function in women with obesity-related infertility, according to some research, but individual responses differ. Bariatric surgery can improve pregnancy outcomes by lowering risks such as gestational diabetes and hypertensive diseases. Women who are considering having a baby after having bariatric surgery should prioritize specialist treatment, nutritional monitoring, and careful supervision to ensure a healthy and successful pregnancy journey.

Bariatric surgery, a weight loss method for chronically obese people, has grown in popularity in recent years. There is evidence that bariatric surgery may help with PCOS in women's health. However, there are also worries regarding how bariatric surgery may influence conception, gestation, and other reproductive functions. In this post, we'll look at how bariatric surgery impacts pregnancy. We'll see how it affects pregnancy outcomes and maternal health.

Does bariatric surgery have an effect on pregnancy outcomes?

Concerns have been raised about potential pregnancy issues following weight loss surgery. Understanding how bariatric surgery may affect maternal and fetal health is critical for those considering pregnancy after surgery.

According to research, bariatric surgery can have a good effect on pregnancy outcomes. Pregnant women who have bariatric surgery may have a lower risk of gestational diabetes, hypertensive disorders, preeclampsia, and large-for-gestational-age kids. Furthermore, after bariatric surgery, women may have better control over their weight increase during pregnancy, which can benefit both the mother and the baby.

What precautions should women take following bariatric surgery during pregnancy?

Certain precautions must be taken by women who have had bariatric surgery and intend to become pregnant in order to have a healthy pregnancy. Addressing dietary needs and any nutrient deficits is critical to supporting mother and fetal well-being. Women who become pregnant following bariatric surgery should receive specialist treatment from healthcare providers who are knowledgeable in managing post-bariatric surgery pregnancies. Regular nutrient monitoring, vitamin and mineral supplementation, and thorough monitoring of weight increase during pregnancy are essential for optimizing results and minimizing potential dangers.

Does bariatric surgery affect the quality of life?

Bariatric surgery is a common weight loss method for severe obesity, affecting patients' physical, psychological, and social lives. While losing weight improves physical health, possible consequences may interfere with regular activities. Psychological advantages include increased self-esteem, yet emotional difficulties may emerge. Changes in appearance and eating habits can have an impact on social interactions, resulting in a variety of social experiences following surgery.

Bariatric surgery is a surgical intervention for severe obesity that has grown in favor as an efficient means of weight loss and overall health improvement. While bariatric surgery has the ability to reduce weight and resolve obesity-related health conditions, it can have a significant impact on the patient's life. In this essay, we will look at the link between bariatric surgery and quality of life, focusing on the physical, psychological, and social aspects.

How does bariatric surgery affect physical quality of life?

Patients' physical well-being and capacity to do everyday tasks are greatly impacted by bariatric surgery, lowering their quality of life. Weight loss by bariatric surgery can enhance mobility, reduce joint discomfort, and resolve obesity-related diseases. However, certain post-surgery issues and adaptations may limit patients' ability to lead an active lifestyle. That is, some people may have temporary post-operative obstacles, such as dietary changes and potential complications, which might have an impact on their quality of life in the near term.

In what ways can bariatric surgery affect psychological quality of life?

Bariatric surgery has a significant impact on patients' psychological well-being and mental health. It improves the psychological well-being of patients. Severe obesity has a significant impact on psychological health, resulting in psychological distress, body image difficulties, and low self-esteem. Significant weight loss frequently results in increased self-esteem and body image, as well as a reduction in symptoms of sadness and anxiety linked with obesity, all of which improves quality of life. However, some patients may face mental difficulties as a result of physical changes and adjusting to their new lifestyle following bariatric surgery, highlighting the significance of post-surgical psychological assistance.

How does bariatric surgery affect the quality of one's social life?

The social quality of life is also affected by bariatric surgery. Post-surgery changes in appearance and eating habits may have an impact on patients' social interactions, relationships, and general sense of belonging. The consequences of bariatric surgery on social interactions can be varied. While some patients may benefit from greater social interactions as a result of increased confidence and well-being, others may struggle with adjusting to social events including food or dealing with reactions from friends and family. Support groups and therapy can be quite beneficial in assisting patients in navigating these changes and maintaining a positive social life.

Below are Some Success Stories of Bariatric Surgery Beneficiaries

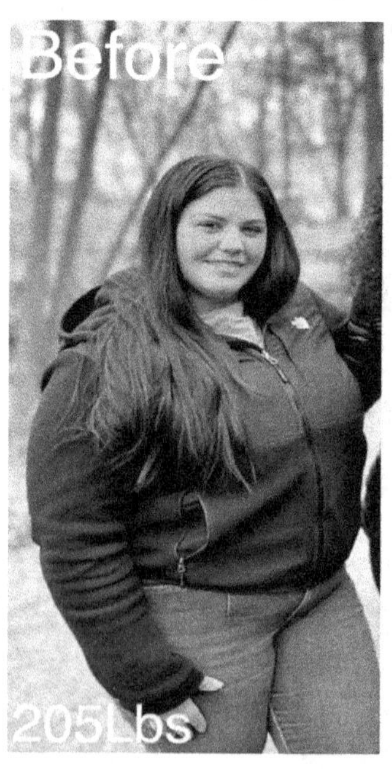

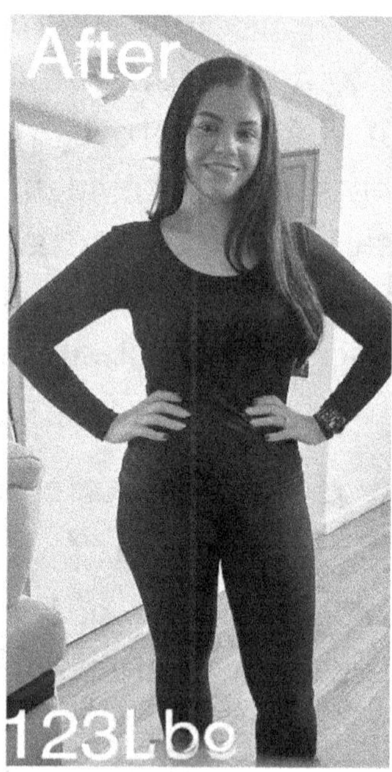

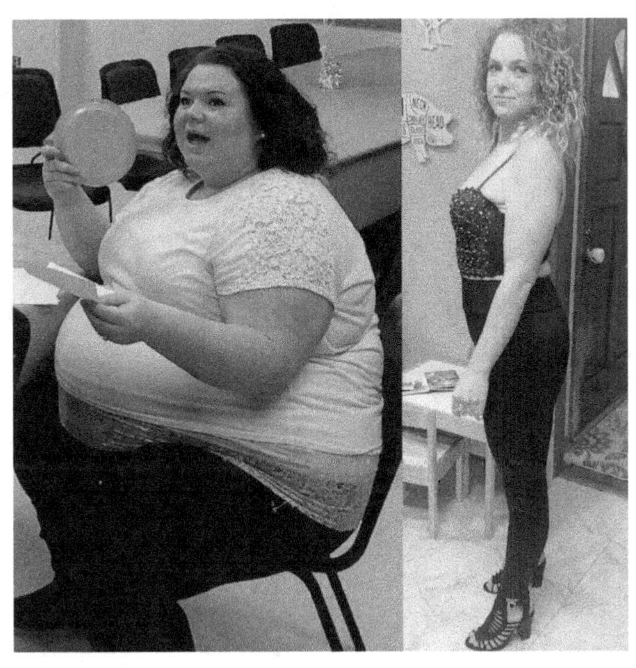

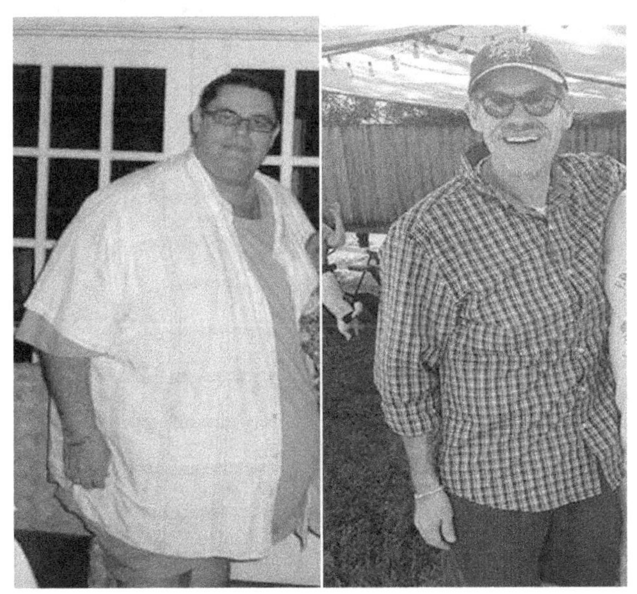